FOGSI EEBR 2025

Ethical Evidence-Based Recommendations

Induction of Labor

Disclaimer

This Ethical Evidence-Based Recommendation (EEBR) document is drafted following a consensus between esteemed FOGSI experts and stakeholders and are based on the scientific evidence available at the time of preparation.

EEBRs should be used for information and educational purposes. They do not replace the need for application of clinical judgment to each individual presentation, or variations based on individual patient and resource setting.

Furthermore, EEBRs do not constitute or imply the endorsement of any of the included technologies, therapies, or techniques by FOGSI.

FOGSI EEBR 2025
Ethical Evidence-Based Recommendations
Induction of Labor

Editor-in-Chief

Sunita Tandulwadkar
MD (Obs and Gyne) FICS (Gyne-Endoscopy) FICOG
President, FOGSI (2025–2026)
Gynecological Endoscopist and ART & IVF Specialist
Head, Department of Obstetrics and Gynecology
Chief, IVF & Endoscopy Center, Ruby Hall Clinic, Pune
Founder and Medical Director
Solo Clinic IVF—A Center for Excellence in Infertility and Endoscopy, Pune
Founder and Medical Director
Solo Stem Cells—A Stem Cell Research and Application Center, Pune
Founder and Director, Alive Regenerative Wellness, Pune, Maharashtra, India

Editors

Manju Puri
MD FRCOG (Hon Causa)
Director Professor
Department of Obstetrics and Gynecology
Lady Hardinge Medical College and
SSK Hospital
New Delhi, India

K Aparna Sharma
MD DNB FICOG MNAMS MSc (Fetal Medicine)
Professor
Department of Obstetrics and Gynecology
All India Institute of Medical Sciences
New Delhi, India

Experts

Ameya C Purandare
MD DNB DGO DGP FCPS FICOG MNAMS
Consultant
Department of Obstetrics and Gynecology
Purandare Hospital, KJ Somaiya Medical
College, Sir HN Reliance Hospital
Mumbai, Maharashtra, India

Uma Wankhede
MD (Obs and Gyne)
Professor and Head
Department of Obstetrics and Gynecology
Government Medical College
Baramati, Maharashtra, India

Convener

Pooja Lodha
DNB (Obs and Gyne)
Fellow, Fetal Medicine, FOGSI-FMF UK Certified
Lead Consultant
Department of Fetal Medicine
Ruby Hall Clinic and Bharati Vidyapeeth University and Hospital, Pune
Director, Kangaroo Cradle, Fetal Care Centre
Pune, Maharashtra, India

JAYPEE BROTHERS MEDICAL PUBLISHERS
The Health Sciences Publisher
New Delhi | London

JAYPEE **Jaypee Brothers Medical Publishers (P) Ltd**

Headquarters

Jaypee Brothers Medical Publishers (P) Ltd
EMCA House, 23/23-B
Ansari Road, Daryaganj
New Delhi 110 002, India
Landline: +91-11-23272143, +91-11-23272703
+91-11-23282021, +91-11-23245672
Email: jaypee@jaypeebrothers.com

Corporate Office

Jaypee Brothers Medical Publishers (P) Ltd
4838/24, Ansari Road, Daryaganj
New Delhi 110 002, India
Phone: +91-11-43574357
Fax: +91-11-43574314
Email: jaypee@jaypeebrothers.com

Overseas Office

JP Medical Ltd.
83, Victoria Street, London
SW1H 0HW (UK)
Phone: +44 20 3170 8910
Fax: +44 (0)20 3008 6180
Email: info@jpmedpub.com

Website: www.jaypeebrothers.com
Website: www.jaypeedigital.com

Inquiries for bulk sales may be solicited at: jaypee@jaypeebrothers.com

FOGSI EEBR 2025—Ethical Evidence-Based Recommendations: Induction of Labor

First Edition: **2025**

ISBN: 978-93-6616-638-4

Printed in India

Contributors

Ameya C Purandare
MD DNB DGO DGP FCPS FICOG MNAMS
Consultant
Department of Obstetrics
and Gynecology
Purandare Hospital, KJ Somaiya Medical
College, Sir HN Reliance Hospital
Mumbai, Maharashtra, India

Anita Yadav
MBBS MS FMAS
Additional Professor
Department of Obstetrics and
Gynecology
All India Institute of Medical Sciences
Nagpur, Maharashtra, India

Anubhuti Rana
MBBS MS (Obs and Gyne)
Associate Professor
Department of Obstetrics and Gynecology
All India Institute of Medical Sciences
New Delhi, India

Apoorva Kulshrestha
MBBS MD
Assistant Professor
Department of Obstetrics and Gynecology
Lady Hardinge Medical College
and SSK Hospital
New Delhi, India

Asmita Kaundal
MBBS MS (Obs and Gyne) DNB MNAMS
FICMCH FICOG IFCPC Diploma in
Advanced ART Diploma in Urogynecology
Diploma in Aesthetic Gynecology
Assistant Professor
Department of Obstetrics
and Gynecology
All India Institute of Medical Sciences
Bilaspur, Himachal Pradesh, India

K Aparna Sharma
MD DNB FICOG MNAMS MSc (Fetal Medicine)
Professor
Department of Obstetrics
and Gynecology
All India Institute of Medical Sciences
New Delhi, India

Manju Puri
MD FRCOG (Hon Causa)
Director Professor
Department of Obstetrics
and Gynecology
Lady Hardinge Medical College
and SSK Hospital
New Delhi, India

Niharika Dhiman
MS MNAMS
Professor
Department of Obstetrics
and Gynecology
Maulana Azad Medical College
New Delhi, India

Prachi Dixit
MBBS MS
Assistant Professor
Department of Obstetrics
and Gynecology
All India Institute of Medical Sciences
Nagpur, Maharashtra, India

Ritu Sharma
MD (Obs and Gynae) FICMCH
Dip CR ACME Fellow
Professor
Department of Obstetrics
and Gynecology
Government Institute of
Medical Sciences
Greater Noida, Uttar Pradesh, India

Shivangni Sinha
MBBS MS
Assistant Professor
Department of Obstetrics and Gynecology
Lady Hardinge Medical College and
SSK Hospital
New Delhi, India

Sunita Tandulwadkar
MD (Obs and Gyne) FICS (Gyne-Endoscopy)
FICOG
President, FOGSI (2025–2026)
Gynecological Endoscopist and
ART & IVF Specialist
Head, Department of Obstetrics
and Gynecology
Chief, IVF & Endoscopy Center
Ruby Hall Clinic, Pune
Founder and Medical Director
Solo Clinic IVF—A Center for Excellence
in Infertility and Endoscopy, Pune
Founder and Medical Director
Solo Stem Cells—A Stem Cell Research
and Application Center, Pune
Founder and Director
Alive Regenerative Wellness
Pune, Maharashtra, India

Tanisha Gupta
MBBS MD (Obs and Gyne)
Senior Resident
Department of Obstetrics and Gynecology
All India Institute of Medical Sciences
New Delhi, India

Uma Wankhede
MD (Obs and Gyne)
Professor and Head
Department of Obstetrics and
Gynecology
Government Medical College
Baramati, Maharashtra, India

Vaishali Korde Nayak
MBBS DGO DNB MNAMS FICOG
Fellow Maternal and Fetal
Medicine (NUH, Singapore)
Professor and Head
Department of Obstetrics
and Gynecology
MIMER Medical College
Pune, Maharashtra, India

Wansalan Karu Shullai
MBBS MS (Obs and Gyne)
Associate Professor
Department of Obstetrics and
Gynecology
North Eastern Indira Gandhi Regional
Institute of Health and Medical
Sciences
Shillong, Meghalaya, India

Preface

Induction of labor (IOL) is a critical component of obstetric care, aimed at safeguarding maternal and neonatal health under specific clinical circumstances. Over recent years, a growing body of evidence has sought to guide practitioners in making informed decisions regarding the timing, methods, and indications for induction, balancing the benefits of intervention against the potential risks. This review presents an ethical and evidence-based approach to induction of labor, providing insights drawn from the latest clinical guidelines and research. This document addresses key clinical questions, offering practical recommendations based on a critical analysis of the available data.

I acknowledge the contributions of a multidisciplinary team of experts in obstetrics and gynecology, whose collaborative efforts have enriched the depth and relevance of this work. I hope that this review serves as a valuable resource for obstetricians to improve maternal and neonatal outcomes through responsible and informed induction practices.

With this series of documents, the Federation of Obstetric and Gynaecological Societies of India (FOGSI) endeavors to provide the practicing obstetricians and gynecologists with the knowledge of advancements in medical science and together with evolving patient needs driving continuous improvements in clinical care.

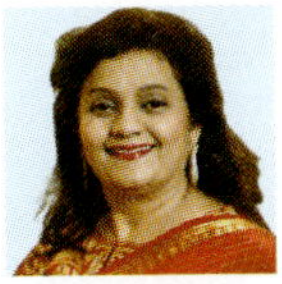

Editor-in-Chief
Sunita Tandulwadkar

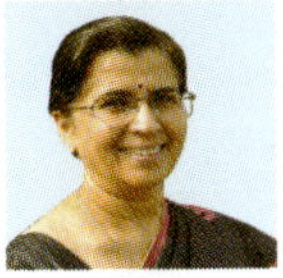

Editor
Manju Puri

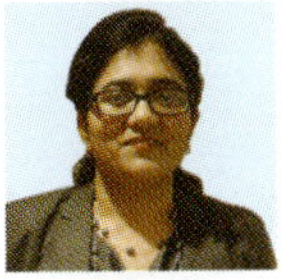

Editor
K Aparna Sharma

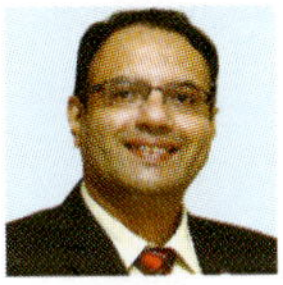

Expert
Ameya C Purandare

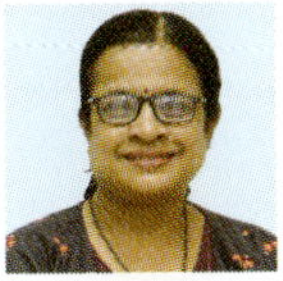

Expert
Uma Wankhede

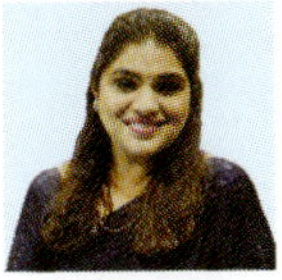

Convener
Pooja Lodha

Contents

Summary of Draft Recommendations

General: Prerequisites, Monitoring, and Complications

- Prerequisites for induction of labor include informed written consent, confirmation of a valid indication for induction, and excluding any contraindication for vaginal birth. This should also include confirming the gestational age, assessment of Bishop score, adequacy of pelvis, and fetal well-being.
- Women undergoing induction of labor, should be monitored by an hourly pulse, 4-hourly temperature, blood pressure and respiratory rate. An abdominal examination must be performed half hourly to monitor frequency and duration of uterine contractions. Fetal heart rate and 4 hourly to assess the descent of fetal head. A vaginal examination is to be done 4 hourly after adequate contractions are established for assessment of the cervical dilatation, effacement, station of the presenting part, and presence or absence of membranes or any caput or molding. A note should be made of any bleeding or leaking per vaginum.
- Use of partogram for monitoring maternal and fetal status and progress of labor is recommended.
- For women undergoing induction of labor with oxytocin or prostaglandin, electronic fetal monitoring (EFM) is desirable. While using mechanical methods, EFM is not mandatory.
- If EFM is not available fetal heart rate must be auscultated every 30 minutes for 1 minute post contraction.
- Induction of labor is associated with complications such as fetal distress, failure of induction and related increase in rate of intervention in the form of instrumental vaginal delivery, caesarean section. In multiparous women undergoing induction of labor with prostaglandins, risk of uterine rupture is higher especially in those with previous scarred uterus.
- Uterine hyperstimulation is seen more with pharmacological methods. It can further lead to complications like rupture of the uterus, amniotic fluid embolism and precipitate labor.
- Cord prolapse can occur if amniotomy is done when the head is high up or not well applied to the cervix.
- Induction of labor is often associated with more pain as compared to spontaneous labor and is more likely to require epidural analgesia.
- Induction may have an adverse impact on the birth experience of women.

Indications and Optimum Gestational Age for Induction of Labor

- Induction of labor may be offered for low-risk pregnant women at ≥39 weeks after a shared decision making.
- In a low-risk women with preterm prelabor rupture of membranes (PPROM) before 34 weeks, expectant management is recommended till 34 weeks of pregnancy in the absence of any intrauterine infection. Expectant management can be offered till 37 weeks of pregnancy after counseling and shared decision making.
- In women with preterm pre-labor rupture of membranes between 34 and 37 weeks of gestation, without any evidence of intrauterine infection, or fetal compromise, either expectant management or induction of labor can be offered until 37 weeks with shared decision making.
- In pregnant women with gestational hypertension, induction of labor is recommended at 37–39 weeks of gestation depending on the severity of hypertension.
- In women with preeclampsia without severe features, induction of labor is recommended at 37 weeks of gestation.
- In a woman with preeclampsia with severe features, induction of labor is to be offered at ≥34 weeks of gestation.
- In a woman with preeclampsia with severe features, less than 34 weeks, expectant management is to be considered till 34 weeks, with a strict watch for any maternal or fetal deterioration, in which case immediate induction of labor is offered.
- Women with well-controlled gestational diabetes mellitus on medical nutrition therapy and no other complication must be offered induction of labor after 39 weeks of gestation.
- In women with well-controlled pregestational diabetes mellitus or gestational diabetes mellitus on oral hypoglycemic agents or insulin, induction of labor should be offered between 38 to 39 weeks of gestation.
- Women with poorly controlled pregestational diabetes mellitus on insulin are offered induction before 37 weeks of gestation. Timing of delivery should be individualized.
- Women with gestational diabetes mellitus or pregestational diabetes mellitus and estimated fetal weight of more than 4000 gm should be offered an elective caesarean section.
- In small for gestational age (SGA) fetuses (estimated fetal weight (EFW) between 3rd and 10th centile and normal Doppler parameters), induction of labor is recommended at 39 weeks if there is no other maternal or fetal indication.
- In FGR fetuses (AC/EFW less than 3rd centile or AC/EFW between 3rd to 10th centile with umbilical artery PI >95th centile), delivery may be planned between 36 to 38 weeks.

- In FGR fetuses with absent or reversed end-diastolic flow in the umbilical artery or abnormal ductus venosus flow, induction of labor is not indicated, and caesarean section should be offered.
- Timing of induction of labor in woman with intrahepatic cholestasis of pregnancy (IHCP) with no other risk factors should be based on concentrations of serum bile acids.
- For women with serum bile acids <40 μmol/L (mild) and no other risk factor, planned birth is offered at 39–40 weeks.
- For serum bile acids between 40–99 μmol/L (moderate) with no other risk factors, induction of labor is offered at 37–38 weeks.
- For serum bile acids ≥100 μmol/L (severe) with no other risk factors, planned birth is offered at 35–36 weeks.
- In women with co-existing risk factors or previous stillbirth due to IHCP timing of offering induction of labor needs to be tailored.
- Induction of labor before 34 weeks is not justified only for IHCP.
- In woman with intrauterine fetal death with (IUFD) with intact membranes and no other complications like preeclampsia, abruption or sepsis, discussion should be done for expectant management versus immediate induction of labor. Woman's preferences should be respected.
- In woman with IUFD with rupture of membranes or any evidence of infection, abruption or preeclampsia, immediate induction of labor is offered.
- In women with uncomplicated dichorionic diamniotic twin pregnancy, induction of labor is offered at 38 weeks of gestation when the first twin is in cephalic presentation.
- In women with uncomplicated monochorionic diamniotic twin pregnancy induction of labor may be offered between 36 to 37 weeks of gestation when first twin is in cephalic presentation.

Cervical Ripening

- Bishop score should be assessed before induction of labor to determine the need for cervical ripening.
- Cervical ripening should be offered when the Bishop score is less than 6.
- Mechanical (balloon catheter) and pharmacological (dinoprostone/PGE2, misoprostol/PGE1) methods are recommended for cervical ripening.
- Dinoprostone (PGE2) gel can be administered either intracervically or intravaginally for cervical ripening.
- For the intracervical route, a dose of 0.5 mg dinoprostone gel is recommended. If the initial dose does not result in Bishop score of ≥6, a second dose may be administered after 6–12 hours. A maximum of three doses (1.5 mg) may be administered within 24 hours.

- For the intravaginal route, a dose of 2–3 mg of dinoprostone tablet may be placed in the posterior fornix of the vagina. If necessary, a repeat dose of 2 mg can be administered after 6–8 hours, with a maximum dose of 6 mg within 24 hours.
- Dinoprostone can be used as a removable controlled release vaginal insert/pessary (10 mg) over 24 hours for cervical ripening.
- Misoprostol (PGE1) is recommended for cervical ripening and can be administered either orally or vaginally.
- The initial dose should be approximately 25 μg, every 2 hours by oral route and every 6 hours by vaginal route
- Higher doses, such as 50 μg every 6 hours, may be considered in certain situations but carry increased risks, including uterine tachysystole and fetal heart rate.
- Mechanical method (balloon catheter) is preferred over prostaglandins for cervical ripening in certain high risk conditions such as grand multipara, SGA or FGR, oligohydramnios or previously scarred uterus compared to prostaglandins.
- Prostaglandins PGE1 and PGE2 by oral route can be used for cervical ripening in women with preterm or pre-labor rupture of membranes.
- Mechanical methods are not recommended in women with ruptured membranes.
- For cervical ripening in women with previous lower segment caesarean section (LSCS), mechanical methods, particularly balloon catheters, are preferred.
- Prostaglandin E2 (dinoprostone) can be used cautiously with close monitoring, but misoprostol should be avoided.
- Sequential use of cervical ripening methods, such as balloon catheters followed by prostaglandins, can be used with caution.
- Simultaneous use of multiple methods is not recommended.
- In cases of unsuccessful cervical ripening, a rest period followed by repeat or an alternate method may be considered after a thorough reassessment of the pregnant woman and the fetus.

Methods of Induction of Labor

- Oxytocin infusion is recommended for induction of labor when the Bishop score ≥6.
- Simultaneous induction with amniotomy and oxytocin, or balloon catheter with oxytocin may be offered to reduce the induction delivery interval.
- Oxytocin should be administered at least 6 hours after inserting vaginal prostaglandin E2, 30 minutes after removing a prostaglandin E2 vaginal

insert, 2 hours after administering oral misoprostol, and 4 hours after inserting vaginal misoprostol.

- Oxytocin should be administered intravenously as an infusion for induction of labor to allow continuous and precise dose control.
- Infusion rates must be recorded in milliunits per minute (mU/min) or drops per minute, with the dilution specified.
- The standard preparation involves diluting 5U of oxytocin in 500 mL (10 mU/mL) of normal saline or Ringer's lactate solution. Both high-dose and low-dose regimens are recommended in primigravida. The low-dose regimen begins at 1–2 mU/min, with incremental increases of 1–2 mU every 30 minutes. The high-dose regimen starts at 4–6 mU/min, with increments of 4–6 mU/min every 15–30 minutes.
- High-dose regimens are not recommended for multigravida and women with a previously scarred uterus.
- A maximum dose of 60 mU/min of oxytocin is recommended for primigravidae while a maximum of 30 mU/min for multigravidae and women with a previous caesarean section.
- For induction of labor, misoprostol may be administered by oral, sublingual, or vaginal route.
- A dose of a 25 μg misoprostol is recommended every 2 hours for oral route and every 6 hours for vaginal route. The dose should be titrated based on the frequency and duration of uterine contractions.
- Misoprostol is not recommended for induction of labor in a scarred uterus.
- Amniotomy is recommended for labor induction when the Bishop score is ≥ 6, and should be used in combination with oxytocin infusion depending on intensity of uterine contraction.
- Due to insufficient evidence, mifepristone is not currently recommended for inducing labor in live pregnancies.
- In women with intrauterine fetal demise, mifepristone in an oral dose of 200–600 mg per day for 1–2 days can be used for cervical ripening.

Definitions

Bishop Score

Bishop score as a scoring system to assess cervical readiness for vaginal delivery and labor induction. It includes cervical dilatation, effacement, consistency, position, and station of fetal head with a possible range of 0–13.

Favorable Cervix

Bishop score is ≥6 is considered favorable as a shorter induction to delivery interval is expected.

Unfavorable Cervix

Bishop score of less than 6 is considered unfavorable as a longer induction to delivery interval is expected and pre-induction cervical ripening is indicated.

Cervical Ripening

The use of pharmacological or other methods to make the cervix favorable (by softening, effacing and/or dilating) for increasing the likelihood of successful outcome of induction of labor.

Induction of Labor

Induction of labor (IOL) refers to the process of artificially stimulating the uterus in order to start labor.

Failed Induction

According to the various guidelines, failed induction is defined as the failure to progress to the active phase of labor after at least 12 hours (range between 12–24 hours) of oxytocin use with ruptured membranes.

Augmentation of Labor

Augmentation of labor is the use of oxytocin to increase the frequency and duration of contractions after the onset of labor.

Tachysystole

Tachysystole is defined as occurrence of more than 5 uterine contractions in 10-minute period averaged over 30 minutes with a normal CTG.

Hypertonus

This is defined as occurrence of a single uterine contraction for more than 2 hours with a normal CTG.

Hyperstimulation

Hyperstimulation is defined as either >5 contractions in 10 minutes averaged over a 30-minute period or contraction lasting more than 2 minutes in duration with fetal heart rate changes.

Adequate Contractions

Adequate uterine contractions are defined as 3–5 contractions in a 10-minute window, each lasting for 30 to 40 seconds. Alternatively, adequate uterine activity is defined when Montevideo units exceed 200 mm Hg.

CHAPTER 1

General: Prerequisites, Monitoring, and Complications

Niharika Dhiman, Vaishali Korde Nayak

PREREQUISITES

Q1. What are the prerequisites for induction of labor?

Draft recommendations: Prerequisites for induction of labor include informed written consent, evaluation of indication of induction, and excluding any contraindication for vaginal birth. This should also include confirming the gestational age, assessment of bishop score, adequacy of pelvis, and fetal well-being.

Evidence summary: According to *WHO guidelines (2011), SLCOG guidelines (2013) and FOGSI-ICOG GCPR (2018)*, the prerequisites & components of preinduction assessment are: Informed written consent, review of maternal history and profile, evaluation for indications and ruling out any contraindications, reliable estimation of gestational age, presentation and fetal weight, maternal pulse, blood pressure, temperature, respiratory rate and findings on abdominal palpation, baseline fetal heart rate pattern by auscultation/electronic fetal monitoring, maternal pelvis assessment and clinical evaluation for possible cephalopelvic, assessment of cervical status using bishop scoring system to predict the likelihood of success and select appropriate method of induction of labor.

As per *NICE guidelines (2021)*, The position of the baby and the condition of the woman should be assessed for suitability for induction. The assessment should include abdominal palpation, bishop score and fetal well-being and absence of significant uterine contractions. The availability of cardiotocography facilities must be ensured.

MONITORING

Q2. How should the patient be monitored during induction of labor?

Draft recommendations:

1. Women undergoing induction of labor, should be monitored by an hourly pulse, 4-hourly temperature, blood pressure and respiratory rate. An abdominal examination must be performed half hourly to monitor frequency and duration of uterine contractions and 4 hourly to determine the descent of fetal head. A vaginal examination is to be done 4 hourly

after adequate contractions are established for assessment of the cervical dilatation, effacement, station of the presenting part, and presence or absence of membranes or any caput or molding. A note should be made of any bleeding or leaking per vaginum.
2. Use of partogram for monitoring maternal and fetal status and progress of labor is recommended.
3. For women undergoing induction of labor with oxytocin or prostaglandin, electronic fetal monitoring (EFM) is desirable. While using mechanical methods, EFM is not mandatory.
4. If EFM is not available fetal heart rate must be auscultated every 30 minutes for 1 minute postcontraction.

Good Practice Point: *Progress of labor must be assessed by abdominal palpation for the descent of head and frequency and duration of contractions. Per vaginal examination must be avoided till adequate uterine contractions are established for more than four hours or earlier if indicated.*

Evidence Summary: All of the available guidelines, suggest that close maternal and fetal monitoring is a must during Induction of labor.

SLCOG guidelines (2013) advise continuous EFM during the administration of oxytocin. As per **NICE (2021)**, once uterine contractions begin with prostaglandins, fetal well-being, and uterine contractions are to be assessed. If the CTG is normal, use intermittent auscultation and if abnormal or there are excessive uterine contractions, continue or restart continuous cardiotocography.

DGGG, OEGGG and SGGG guidelines (2020) do not recommend CTG examinations mandatorily in induction with mechanical methods as they lead to cervical ripening through endogenous release of prostaglandins. CTG examinations are recommended in cases of vaginal bleeding or other abnormalities.

FOGSI-ICOG GCPR (2018) recommends monitoring the progress of labor using a partograph.

NICE guidelines (2023) guidelines advise half-hourly documentation of the frequency of contractions, hourly pulse 4-hourly temperature, blood pressure and respiratory rate, auscultation of fetal heart rate for a minimum of 1 minute immediately after a contraction if not on EFM in the first stage of labor. It recommends 4-hourly vaginal examination to determine the station and the position of the presenting part, cervical effacement, cervical dilatation, presence or absence of membranes and any caput or molding.

COMPLICATIONS

Q3. What are the complications of induction of labor?

Draft recommendations:

1. Induction of labor is associated with complications such as fetal distress, failure of induction and an increased rate of intervention in the form of instrumental vaginal delivery, caesarean section. In multiparous women undergoing induction of labor with prostaglandins, risk of uterine rupture is higher especially in those with previous scarred uterus.
2. Uterine hyperstimulation is seen more with pharmacological methods. It can further lead to complications like rupture of the uterus, amniotic fluid embolism and precipitate labor.
3. Cord prolapse can occur if amniotomy is done when the head is high up or not well applied to the cervix.
4. Induction of labor is often associated with more pain as compared to spontaneous labor and are more likely to require epidural analgesia.
5. induction may have an adverse impact on the birth experience of women.

Evidence summary: As per *WHO guidelines (2011), SLCOG guidelines (2013)* and *NICE guidelines(2023),* induction of labor is associated with complications such as uterine hyperstimulation, cord prolapse, uterine rupture and increased pain during labor. According to *NICE guidelines(2023),* mechanical methods are less likely to cause hyperstimulation than pharmacological methods. Hyperstimulation caused by misoprostol may be more difficult to reverse. As induction is associated with more pain, epidural analgesia should be provided. Multiparous women induced with prostaglandin had an increased risk of uterine rupture compared with nulliparous women (adjusted odds ratio [OR], 3.33 [95% confidence interval (CI), 1.38–8.04]; $p < 0.007$). Multiparous women with no previous caesarean section (CS) induced with prostaglandin had more than three times higher risk of uterine rupture (crude OR, 3.55 [95% Cl, 48–8.53]; $p = 0.005$) compared with nulliparous women. Women undergoing induction of labor with misoprostol (PGE1) administered vaginally are at higher risk of meconium staining of liquor especially if the cervix is unfavorable.

CHAPTER 2

Indications and Optimum Gestational Age for Induction of Labor

Asmita Kaundal, Prachi Dixit, Ritu Sharma

LOW-RISK PREGNANCY

Q1. In low-risk pregnant women what is the optimum gestational age (39-42 weeks) for induction of labor (IOL) to optimize maternal and perinatal outcomes?

Draft recommendations: Induction of labor may be considered in low-risk women after 39 weeks following a shared decision making.

Research gap: There is a need to generate evidence on the ideal time for induction of labor among low risk pregnant women and compare outcomes in inductions performed at 39, 40 and 41 weeks.

Evidence summary: In low-risk pregnancies, many studies have compared outcomes of induction of labor at various gestational ages ranging from 39 to 42 weeks' of gestation versus expectant management. *ACOG guidelines (2009)* states that there is no role of induction of labor at 39 weeks without any maternal or fetal indication. *SLCOG guidelines (2013) and Queensland guidelines (2022) and WHO guidelines (2022*) on induction of labor in women with prolonged pregnancy recommend that IOL should be offered to women at or beyond 41 weeks. *SOGC guidelines (2017) and DGGG, OEGGG and SGGG guidelines (2020)* recommend that women should be offered induction between 41+0 to 42+0 weeks, as it results in a decrease in perinatal mortality without any increase in the risk of cesarean section. However, for waiting beyond 41 weeks antenatal monitoring should include at least a NST and an assessment of amniotic fluid volume. *NICE guidelines (2021)* emphasize on giving all uncomplicated pregnancies every opportunity to go in spontaneous labor till 42 weeks but suggest a discussion with the woman that the chances of neonatal ICU (NICU) admission, neonatal death and cesarean section increase if pregnancy is continued after 41 weeks' of gestation and that induction of labor from 41+0 weeks may reduce these risks. *FOGSI-ICOG GCPR (2018)* guidelines recommends that induction of labor in low risk pregnancies can be offered any time after 39 weeks.

ARRIVE trial (2018) was a randomized trial of induction versus expectant management on more than 6000 low-risk nulliparas. Women were randomly assigned to labor induction or expectant management group at

39 weeks' gestation. The rate of severe neonatal morbidity or death did not differ between the two cohorts. However, the cesarean delivery rate in the induction arm was significantly lower than that in the expectantly managed cohort (18.6 versus 22.2%), respectively. Rates of chorioamnionitis, postpartum hemorrhage, and peripartum infection were not significantly different.

A meta-analysis by Sotiriadis A et al. (2019) on elective induction at 39 weeks concluded that elective induction of labor in uncomplicated singleton pregnancy at 39 weeks' gestation is not associated with maternal or perinatal complications and may reduce the need for cesarean section, risk of hypertensive disorder of pregnancy and need for neonatal respiratory support. Similarly, another *meta-analysis of randomized trials by Saccone G et al. (2019)* on induction of labor at full term in pregnant women concluded that induction at 39 weeks was not associated with an increased risk of cesarean section. However, they did not find any difference in other adverse neonatal outcomes.

PRELABOR RUPTURE OF MEMBRANES

Q1. Does induction of labor versus expectant management in women with preterm prelabor rupture of membranes (PPROM) improve maternal and fetal outcome?

Draft recommendations:

1. In a low-risk women with preterm prelabor rupture of membranes (PPROM) before 34 weeks, without any evidence of intrauterine infection, expectant management is recommended till 34 weeks of pregnancy. In these women, without any evidence of intrauterine infection, further expectant management can be offered till 37 weeks of pregnancy after counseling and shared decision making.
2. In women with preterm prelabor rupture of membranes between 34 and 37 weeks' of gestation, without evidence of intrauterine infection, or fetal compromise, either expectant management or induction of labor can be offered until 37 weeks with shared decision making.

Evidence summary: PPROM is defined as rupture of membranes prior to 37 weeks of pregnancy. PPROM is often complicated by preterm birth, chorioamnionitis, increased maternal and perinatal morbidity and mortality. Most of the guidelines recommend deciding on induction of labor after balancing the risk of prematurity with sepsis. *SLCOG guidelines (2013)* recommend that women with PPROM before 34 weeks of gestation should be offered induction after completion of 34 weeks. *FOGSI-ICOG-GCPR (2018)* states that if PPROM occurs after 34 weeks, the plan for induction should be made after discussing the risks of sepsis to the woman and to the baby, complications of preterm birth and availability of neonatal intensive care facilities. If preterm prelabor rupture of membranes occurs after the period of viability but before 34 weeks induction of labor should not be carried out before 34 weeks, unless there are additional indications (chorioamnionitis or fetal compromise) (4). *Polish guidelines (2017), and DGGG, OEGGG, and SGGG 2020 guidelines* recommend induction of labor by 37 + 0 week of gestation in PPROM if there are no signs of chorioamnionitis (12,22). *NICE guidelines (2021) and FIGO guidelines (2023)* state that, if a woman has PPROM, induction of labor should not be done before 34+0 weeks unless there are additional indications (for example, infection or fetal compromise). Expectant management should be offered till 37+0 week. If a woman has PPROM after 34+0 weeks, but before 37+0 weeks, discuss the options of expectant management or induction of labor until 37+0 weeks. When making a shared decision, take into consideration the risks of maternal sepsis, need for cesarean birth, risks of neonatal sepsis and prematurity, availability of neonatal intensive care facilities, the woman's individual circumstances and her preferences.

Q2. Does induction of labor in women with prelabor rupture of membranes (PROM) at ≥37 weeks' of gestation, improve maternal and fetal outcomes as compared to expectant management?

Draft recommendations:

1. In women with PROM ≥37 weeks' of gestation with no evidence of intrauterine infection, or fetal compromise, either immediate induction of labor or expectant management for up to 24 hours may be offered after adequate counseling and a shared decision.
2. In women with PROM with intrauterine infection, induction of labor is recommended regardless of the gestational age.

Evidence summary: *WHO guidelines (2011), Polish guidelines (2017), and FOGSI-ICOG GCPR (2018)* recommend IOL for women with PROM at ≥37 weeks, as it decreases the risk of maternal and neonatal complications. *SLCOG guidelines (2013)* recommend delayed induction of labor after 24 hours in the absence of evidence fetal compromise or maternal infection. *NICE guidelines (2021), FIGO guidelines (2023) and SOGC guidelines (2023),* recommend that in women with PROM at term offer a choice of expectant management for up to 24 hours, or induction of labor as soon as possible.

HYPERTENSIVE DISORDERS IN PREGNANCY

Q1. In women with gestational hypertension does induction of labor at 37 weeks improve maternal and fetal outcomes compared to expectant management?

Draft recommendations: In pregnant women with gestational hypertension, induction of labor is recommended at 37–39 weeks' of gestation depending on the severity of hypertension.

Evidence summary: Hypertensive disorders of pregnancy are associated with adverse maternal and fetal outcomes if not attended timely. The management depends on the severity of hypertensive disorder and gestational age. *As per ACOG guidelines (2020), SOGC guidelines (2022), DGGG, OEGGG and SGGG guidelines (2020),* in women with gestational hypertension delivery rather than expectant management upon diagnosis is recommended. *NICE guidelines (2023)* recommends that in women with gestational hypertension with blood pressure lower than 160/110 mm Hg, induction of labor should not be offered at 37 weeks, unless there are other medical indications. In those with blood pressure lower than 160/110 mm Hg after 37 weeks, timing of birth, and maternal and fetal indications for birth should be agreed between the woman and the obstetrician.

Q2. In women with preeclampsia without severe features, does induction of labor at 37 weeks, improve maternal and fetal outcomes compared to expectant management?

Draft recommendations: In women with preeclampsia without severe features, induction of labor is recommended at 37 weeks' of gestation.

Evidence summary: Hypertensive disorders of pregnancy are associated with adverse maternal and fetal outcomes if not attended timely. The management depends on the severity of hypertensive disorder and gestational age. As per *ACOG guidelines (2020), SOGC guidelines (2022), DGGG, OEGGG and SGGG guidelines (2020)* in women with preeclampsia without severe features at or beyond 37 0/7 weeks' of gestation, delivery rather than expectant management upon diagnosis is recommended. *NICE guidelines (2023)* recommends that in women with preeclampsia without severe features initiate birth at 37 weeks.

Q3. In women with preeclampsia with severe features, does induction of labor improve maternal and fetal outcomes compared to expectant management?

Draft recommendations:

1. In a woman with preeclampsia with severe features, induction of labor is to be offered at ≥34 weeks' of gestation.
2. In a woman with preeclampsia with severe features, less than 34 weeks, expectant management is to be considered till 34 weeks, with a strict watch for any maternal or fetal deterioration, in which case immediate induction of labor is offered.

Evidence summary: All the guidelines unanimously recommend that in severe preeclampsia before 34 weeks' of gestation expectant management is followed with strict monitoring till 34 weeks. If any signs of maternal or fetal worsening are seen during expectant management that delivery is recommended either by induction of labor or cesarean section. As per *FOGSI-ICOG-GCPR (2018) and ACOG guidelines (2020),* delivery is recommended when preeclampsia with severe features is diagnosed at or beyond 34 0/7 weeks' of gestation, after maternal stabilization. Delivery should not be delayed for the administration of steroids in the late preterm period. *DGGG, OEGGG and SGGG guidelines (2020)* recommendations for women with preeclampsia between 34 to 37 weeks state that maternal morbidity is lower when induced at 34 weeks, however infant morbidity may be higher, particularly before 37 weeks. *SOGC guidelines (2022)* recommends that at 34–35 weeks' gestation, initiation of delivery should be discussed, as it decreases maternal but increases neonatal risk, particularly if antenatal corticosteroids are not prescribed. At 36–37 weeks gestation, initiation of delivery should be considered. At 37 weeks' gestation or later, initiation of delivery is recommended.

HYPERGLYCEMIA IN PREGNANCY

Q1. Does induction of labor in women with well-controlled gestational diabetes mellitus (GDM) on medical nutrition therapy (MNT) improve maternal and fetal outcomes compared to expectant management?

Draft recommendations: Women with well-controlled gestational diabetes mellitus on medical nutrition therapy and no other complication must be offered induction of labor after 39 weeks' of gestation.

Evidence summary: According to *ACOG guidelines (2018),* the timing of delivery in women with well controlled GDM on MNT should not be before 39 weeks of gestation, unless otherwise indicated. In such women, expectant management up to 40+6 weeks of gestation in the setting of indicated antepartum testing is generally appropriate. *Ministry of Health and Family Welfare India Technical operational guidelines (2018)* and *FOGSI-ICOG GCPR (2018)* recommend scheduling induction of labor at or after 39 weeks pregnancy in women with GDM well controlled on MNT. *SOGC guidelines (2019)* states that pregnant women with GDM should be offered induction between 38-40 weeks of gestation depending on their glycemic control and other co-morbidities. *NICE guidelines (2020)* recommends women with gestational diabetes to give birth no later than 40 weeks plus 6 days by induced labor. *Queensland guidelines (2021)* recommend that if GDM is well managed with MNT wait for spontaneous labor and consider birth from 38+0 to 39+0 weeks if there is suspected fetal macrosomia or any other complications.

Q2. Does induction of labor in women with well controlled pregestational diabetes mellitus/gestational diabetes mellitus on medications improve maternal and fetal outcomes compared to expectant management?

Draft recommendations: In women with well-controlled pregestational diabetes mellitus or gestational diabetes mellitus on oral hypoglycemic agents or insulin, induction of labor should be offered between 38 to 39 weeks' of gestation.

Evidence summary: *ACOG guidelines (2018) and Queensland guidelines (2021)* recommend that for women with well-controlled GDM on medications, delivery is recommended at 39+0 to 39+6 weeks of gestation. *FOGSI-ICOG-GCPR (2018)* recommends induction of labor at 38 weeks of gestation if diabetes is controlled on insulin/oral hypoglycemics. *NICE guidelines (2020)* advises pregnant women with type 1 or type 2 diabetes to have an elective birth by induction of labor between 37 and 38+6 week.

Q3. Does induction of labor in women with poorly controlled pregestational diabetes improve maternal and fetal outcomes as compared to expectant management?

Draft recommendations: Women with poorly controlled pregestational diabetes mellitus on Insulin must be offered induction before 37 weeks of gestation. Timing of delivery should be individualized.

Evidence summary: *FOGSI-ICOG GCPR (2018)* states that management of women with uncontrolled diabetes should be individualized. *Ministry of Health and Family Welfare India Technical operational guidelines (2018)* advice that in pregnant women with poorly controlled GDM, those with risk factors like hypertensive disorder of pregnancy, previous still birth and other complications should be delivered earlier. The timing of delivery should be individualized. As per *NICE (2020),* elective birth should be considered before 37 weeks for women with type 1 or type 2 diabetes who have metabolic or other maternal or fetal complications.

Q4. Is elective cesarean delivery preferred over induction of labor in women with gestational diabetes mellitus with ultrasound (USG) diagnosed fetal macrosomia?

Draft recommendations: Women with gestational diabetes mellitus or pregestational diabetes mellitus and estimated fetal weight of more than 4,000 g should be offered an elective cesarean section.

Evidence summary: When estimated fetal weight is more than 4,500 g then risks of perinatal birth trauma and shoulder dystocia, including severe perineal tears, fractures to the baby and brachial plexus injuries are high. *According to ACOG guidelines (2018)* and *Queensland guidelines (2021),* women with GDM should be counseled regarding the risks and benefits of a scheduled cesarean delivery when the estimated fetal weight is 4,500 g or more. *Ministry of Health and Family Welfare India Technical operational guidelines (2018)* advice that in case of fetal macrosomia (estimated fetal weight >4 kg) consideration should be given for elective cesarean section at 39 weeks. *NICE guidelines (2020)* mentions that for pregnant women with diabetes who have an ultrasound-diagnosed macrosomic fetus, explain the risks and benefits of vaginal birth, induction of labor and cesarean section and make a shared decision.

FETAL GROWTH RESTRICTION

Q1. Does induction of labor in women with fetal growth restriction (FGR) improve perinatal outcome compared to expectant management?

Draft recommendations:

1. In small for gestational age (SGA) fetuses (estimated fetal weight (EFW) between 3rd and 10th centile with normal Doppler parameters), induction of labor is recommended at 39 weeks if there is no other maternal or fetal compromise.
2. In FGR fetuses (AC/EFW less than 3rd centile or AC/EFW between 3rd to 10th centile with umbilical artery PI>95th centile), delivery may be planned between 36 to 38 weeks.
3. In FGR fetuses with absent or reversed end-diastolic flow in the umbilical artery or abnormal ductus venosus flow, induction of labor is not indicated, and cesarean section should be performed.

Good practice point: *Induction of labor should not be offered before 38 weeks in fetuses with EFW between 3–10th centile with normal umbilical artery Doppler and abnormal CPR (<5th centile).*

Evidence summary: FGR is an important cause of stillbirth and increased neonatal morbidity and mortality. Timing of delivery is challenging as a balance has to be set between prematurity and risk of stillbirth. The recommendation on timing of delivery is largely influenced by Growth Restriction Intervention Trial (GRIT) and Disproportionate Intrauterine Growth Intervention Trial At Term (DIGITAT) for late onset FGR and by Trial of Umbilical and Fetal Flow in Europe (TRUFFLE) for early-onset FGR.

ISUOG guidelines (2020), FIGO guidelines (2021), RCOG guidelines (2024), agree that the decision for induction of labor in a fetus with growth restriction should be individualized based on period of gestation and presence or absence of fetal compromise (abnormal Doppler parameters).

ISUOG (2020) states that in SGA fetuses (EFW between 3rd and 10th centile with normal Doppler parameters), delivery should be planned from 38 + 0 weeks and the pregnancy should not exceed 39 + 0 weeks of gestation.

RCOG (2024) recommends that in fetuses with EFW between 3rd and 10th centile with normal Doppler parameters) other features like maternal medical conditions or concerns regarding fetal movements or fetal compromise (a diagnosis of FGR based on Doppler assessment, fetal growth velocity or a concern on cardiotocography, must be present to recommend birth prior to 39+0 weeks.

ISUOG (2020) recommends that for fetuses with abdominal circumference (AC)/EFW less than 3rd centile or AC/ EFW between 3rd to 10th centile and an umbilical artery Doppler more than 95th centile delivery is recommended between 36+0 to 37+6 weeks of gestation. Delivery should be conducted between 38+0 to 39+0 if there is an evidence cerebral blood flow redistribution or any other feature of FGR.

Polish guidelines (2017) and RCOG guidelines (2024) state that, induction of labor for FGR is recommended after 37 weeks due to an increased risk of intrauterine fetal death after this gestation. *FIGO guidelines (2021)* recommends that in case of isolated estimated fetal weight <3rd percentile with no additional abnormalities, delivery may be deferred until 36–38 weeks.

FOGSI-ICOG-GCPR (2018), NICE guidelines (2021), FIGO guidelines (2021) recommend against induction of labor in FGR with absent or reversed end-diastolic velocity (AREDV) and the pregnancy should be terminated (with delay depending on the Doppler finding) by cesarean section. *FIGO guidelines (2021)* recommends that cesarean delivery should be the first choice in cases of fetal growth restriction associated with umbilical artery flow with AREDV.

INTRAHEPATIC CHOLESTASIS OF PREGNANCY

Q1. Does induction of labor versus expectant management in women with Intrahepatic cholestasis of pregnancy (IHCP) improve fetal and maternal outcome?

Draft recommendations:

1. Timing of induction of labor in woman with intrahepatic cholestasis of pregnancy (IHCP) with no other risk factors should be based on concentrations of serum bile acids.
2. For women with serum bile acids <40 μmol/L (mild) and no other risk factor, planned birth should be offered at 39–40 weeks.
3. For serum bile acids between 40–99 μmol/L (moderate) with no other risk factors, induction of labor should be offered at 37–38 weeks.
4. For serum bile acids ≥100 μmol/L (severe) with no other risk factors, planned birth should be offered at 35–36 weeks.
5. In women with co-existing risk factors or previous stillbirth due to IHCP timing of offering induction of labor needs to be tailored.
6. Induction of labor before 34 weeks is not justified only for IHCP.

Evidence summary: IHCP affects around 1–2% of the women of Indian-Asian origin mostly in third trimester of pregnancy. It is associated with risk of still birth which remain the subject of concern for women diagnosed with IHCP. Depending upon the level of serum bile acids IHCP is categorized into mild (serum bile acid 19–39 μmol/L), moderate (40–99 μmol/L) and severe (≥100 μmol/L). All the guidelines recommend that the timing of induction of labor in women with IHCP should be based on concentrations of serum bile acids. As the risk of still birth in women with serum bile acid below 100 μmol/L is comparable to the risk in general population, most of the guidelines opine on early induction of labor in women with serum bile acid ≥100μmol/L. For mild and moderate IHCP, timing for induction of labor varies through guideline and most recommend induction of labor by 38-40 weeks. *Polish guidelines (2017)* recommends labor induction after 38 weeks' of gestation in mild ICP, after 36 weeks in moderate IHCP and after 34 weeks of gestation in severe IHCP. *DGGG, OEGGG, SGGG guidelines (2020)* recommends that induction of labor at 37 weeks' of gestation if the pregnant woman has mild/moderate IHCP and between 34 + 0 and 36 + 6 weeks' of gestation in severe IHCP. *SMFM guidelines (2021)* recommends that induction of labor between 36 and 39+0 weeks of gestation for women with mild/moderate IHCP and at 36+6 weeks in women with severe IHCP.

Society of obstetric medicine Australia and New Zealand guidelines (2023) and RCOG guidelines (2022) advises induction of labor by 40 weeks in mild ICP, by 38–39 weeks gestation in moderate ICP and at 35–36 weeks in severe ICP. *FIGO guidelines (2023)* recommends induction at 39 weeks in mild IHCP, at 37–38 weeks in moderate IHCP and at 35–36 weeks in severe IHCP.

INTRAUTERINE FETAL DEATH

Q1. Does induction of labor in women with intrauterine fetal death (IUFD) improve maternal outcomes as compared to expectant management?

Draft recommendations:

1. In woman with intrauterine fetal death with (IUFD) with intact membranes, no evidence of infection and no other additional complications like preeclampsia, abruption or sepsis, discussion should be done for expectant management versus immediate induction of labor. Woman's preferences should be respected.
2. In woman with IUFD with rupture of membranes or any evidence of infection, abruption or preeclampsia, immediate induction of labor should be offered.

Evidence summary: Diagnosis of IUFD is traumatic for both the couple and the caregiver. On one hand woman might need some time to grieve over her loss, on the other hand delaying delivery might lead to increased anxiety in the woman. Risk of complications is also low within first 48 hours. *RCOG guidelines (2010) and FOGSI-ICOG-GCPR (2018)* recommend that, in an otherwise low risk woman diagnosed with intrauterine fetal death with intact membranes, discussion should be done regarding immediate induction of labor versus expectant management for another 48 hours. However, if there is evidence of rupture of membranes, infection or bleeding it is recommended to offer immediate induction of labor or cesarean birth as per the maternal condition. *NICE guidelines (2021), ACOG guidelines and SLCOG guidelines (2013)* recommend that in IUFD, labor and birth should take into account mother's preferences, her medical condition and previous intrapartum history. If induction is delayed for more than 48 hours, woman should have testing for disseminated coagulation failure twice a week). Women contemplating prolonged expectant management should be advised that the value of postmortem examination of the still born fetus may be reduced.

TWIN PREGNANCY

Q1. In pregnant women with dichorionic diamniotic twin pregnancy, does induction of labor as compared to expectant management improve perinatal outcome?

Draft recommendations: In women with uncomplicated dichorionic diamniotic twin pregnancy, induction of labor should be offered at 38 weeks' of gestation when the first twin in cephalic presentation.

Evidence summary: *FOGSI-ICOG-GCPR (2018) and DGGG, OEGGG and SGGG guidelines (2020)* state that in uncomplicated twin pregnancy, where there are no contraindications to vaginal delivery, induction of labor at 37 weeks is advisable. *ACOG guidelines (2021)* recommends that women with uncomplicated dichorionic-diamniotic twin gestations can undergo delivery at 38+0 to 38+6 weeks' of gestation. *SOGC guidelines (2022)* recommends that women with an uncomplicated dichorionic twin pregnancy should be offered elective delivery at 37–38 weeks' gestation. *NICE guidelines (2024)* recommends discussing with woman with a dichorionic diamniotic twin pregnancy that continuing the pregnancy beyond 37+6 weeks increases the risk of fetal death.

Q2. In pregnant women with uncomplicated monochorionic diamniotic twin pregnancy, does induction of labor improve perinatal outcome as compared to expectant management?

Draft recommendations: In women with uncomplicated monochorionic diamniotic twin pregnancy induction of labor may be offered between 36 to 37 weeks' of gestation when first twin in cephalic presentation.

Evidence summary: *ACOG guidelines (2021)* says that women with uncomplicated monochorionic-diamniotic twin gestations can undergo delivery between 34+0 weeks and 37+6 weeks of gestation. **S***OGC guidelines (2023)* recommends that monochorionic twins without complications should be delivered between 36 and 37 weeks gestation. *NICE guidelines (2024)* recommends that women with uncomplicated monochorionic diamniotic twin pregnancy must be explained that continuing the pregnancy beyond 36+6 weeks increases the risk of fetal death.

CHAPTER 3

Cervical Ripening

Anita Yadav, Wansalan Karu Shullai, Shivangni Sinha

INDICATION

Q1. For a pregnant woman planned for induction of labor, when should preinduction cervical ripening be offered?

Draft recommendations:

1. Bishop score should be assessed to determine the need for cervical ripening.
2. Cervical ripening should be offered when the Bishop score is less than 6.

Evidence summary: Various guidelines provide a comprehensive framework for determining when cervical ripening should be offered, emphasizing the role of Bishop score and clinical evaluation. The *FOGSI-ICOG GCPR (2018) and NICE guidelines (2021)* recommend using the Bishop score to guide the choice between pharmacological and mechanical methods for induction of labor. A Bishop score of <6 indicates the need for cervical ripening methods, while a score of ≥6 suggests a favorable cervix with a higher likelihood of spontaneous labor or a better response to induction interventions. The *SOGC guidelines (2023)* recommend using and documenting the Bishop score to assess the need for cervical ripening and initiating cervical ripening when the Bishop score is less than 7.

METHODS

Q1. What are the various methods available for cervical ripening?

Draft recommendations: Mechanical (balloon catheter) and pharmacological (dinoprostone/PGE2 and misoprostol/PGE1) methods are recommended for cervical ripening.

Evidence summary: The evidence supports the use of both mechanical and pharmacological methods for cervical ripening, with various guidelines recommending specific approaches based on their safety, efficacy, and suitability in different clinical scenarios. *SOGC guidelines (2023)* recommends balloon catheter as first-line method for cervical ripening whenever feasible, as they are safe and effective, including in an outpatient setting and for induction of labor in women with previous cesarean section. It also recommends that prostaglandin E2 vaginal gel or insert can be used for cervical ripening to achieve safe and effective cervical ripening. It further recommends that prostaglandin and balloon catheters may be used concurrently for cervical ripening. According to *FOGSI-ICOG GCPR (2018),* both dinoprostone gel (0.5 mg dinoprostone) and dinoprostone vaginal pessary (10 mg embedded in a mesh) have equal efficacy and result in a significantly lower cesarean delivery rate and an increased proportion of vaginal deliveries within 24 hours as compared to expectant management. It also recommends the use of transcervical balloon catheter as a preferred choice of cervical ripening in cases of scarred uterus provided there are no signs of infection.

Queensland guidelines (2022) recommend use of mechanical methods (balloon catheter) and pharmacological agents like dinoprostone (prostaglandin E2) vaginal gel and vaginal slow-release pessary for cervical ripening in unfavorable cervix.

Misoprostol (PGE1) is widely recommended for cervical ripening in various clinical guidelines. *ACOG guidelines (2009)* suggests its use intravaginally, orally, or sublingually, with an initial dose of 25 mcg every 3-6 hours, while *WHO guidelines (2011)* recommend 25 μg oral dose every 2 hours or low-dose vaginal misoprostol every 6 hours. Despite its efficacy, **FOGSI-ICOG GCPR (2018)** notes that misoprostol is not approved for labor induction in India, while *SLCOG guidelines (2013) and Queensland guidelines (2022)* also advise against its use in cases with a live fetus. **SOGC guidelines (2023)** recommend misoprostol for cervical ripening when the fetus has a normal electronic fetal heart rate tracing, but suggest caution in potentially compromised fetuses.

Q2. What are the recommended routes and doses of dinoprostone (PGE2) for cervical ripening?

Draft recommendations:

1. Dinoprostone (PGE2) gel can be administered either intracervically or intravaginally for cervical ripening.
2. For the intracervical route, a dose of 0.5 mg dinoprostone gel is recommended. If the initial dose does not result in adequate cervical change, a second dose may be administered after 6–12 hours. The maximum of three doses (1.5 mg) may be administered within 24 hours.
3. For the intravaginal route, a dose of 2–3 mg of dinoprostone tablet should be placed in the posterior fornix of the vagina. If necessary, a repeat dose of 2 mg can be administered after 6–8 hours, with a maximum dose of 6 mg within 24 hours.
4. Dinoprostone can be used as a removable controlled release vaginal insert/pessary (10 mg) over 24 hours for cervical ripening.

Evidence summary: The dosage and administration techniques vary across different guidelines, but all emphasize the importance of careful monitoring to mitigate the risk of uterine hyperstimulation.

The *ACOG guidelines (2009) and FOGSI-ICOG GCPR (2018)* both recommend the use of dinoprostone (PGE2) for cervical ripening, with two main forms available: intracervical gel and vaginal inserts/pessaries. Both guidelines suggest that intracervical dinoprostone gel (0.5 mg) can be administered, with repeat dosing allowed after 6–12 hours if there is inadequate cervical change. The maximum recommended dosage is three doses within a 24-hour period. Similarly, the vaginal pessary, containing 10 mg of dinoprostone, releases the drug at a rate of approximately 0.3 mg per hour over 24 hours. The pessary should be removed either at the end of the 24-hour dosing period or once the labor is established, whichever occurs first. If the membranes rupture after pessary insertion, it does not necessitate removal of the pessary. *WHO guidelines (2011)* recommend using low doses of vaginal prostaglandins for labor induction. Vaginal prostaglandin E2 (PGE2) gel is preferred over vaginal PGE2 tablets and suppositories/pessaries, as it is associated with a lower risk of uterine hyperstimulation. Additionally, vaginal PGE2 gel is more effective than intracervical PGE2 gel for cervical ripening, reducing the likelihood of failed vaginal births within 24 hours. However, while vaginal PGE2 carries a higher risk of uterine hyperstimulation with fetal heart rate changes, it does not significantly increase adverse maternal or perinatal outcomes. *SLCOG guidelines (2013)* recommend the use of prostaglandin E2 (PGE2) for inducing labor. The recommended routes are vaginal gel, tablet, or controlled release pessary. The dosages are 3 mg for vaginal tablets and 0.5 mg for vaginal gel. A second dose may be considered after a minimum interval of 6 hours from the first dose, depending on the change in Bishop score, fetal condition, and frequency of contractions. The intracervical route does not offer increased efficacy. All preparations carry a risk of hyperstimulation, and combined use with oxytocin is particularly dangerous. The *Polish guidelines (2017)* recommend using prostaglandin E2 (PGE2) for cervical ripening. The recommended routes are vaginal gel (0.5 mg/3 g) and a vaginal delivery system (0.005 g/12 hours). The *Queensland guidelines (2022)* recommend the use of 2 mg dose dinoprostone vaginal gel inserted high into the posterior fornix for cervical ripening in nulliparous women and 1 mg dose for multiparous women. For the vaginal pessary, a single dose of 10 mg dose is positioned transversely in the posterior fornix, and reassessment should occur at least 12 hours post-insertion. It may be used for up to 24 hours. If the gel is used, up to three doses can be administered, with at least six hours between doses.

Q3. What are the recommended routes and doses of misoprostol (PGE1) for cervical ripening?

Draft recommendations:

1. Misoprostol (PGE1) is recommended for cervical ripening and can be administered either orally or vaginally.
2. The initial dose should be approximately 25 µg, every 2 hours by oral route and every 6 hours by vaginal route.
3. Higher doses, such as 50 µg every 6 hours, may be considered in certain situations but carry increased risks, including uterine tachysystole and fetal heart rate.

Evidence summary: The evidence supports the use of misoprostol (PGE1) for cervical ripening, with several guidelines recommending its administration through oral or vaginal routes, typically at a low dose of 25 µg. *ACOG guidelines (2009), WHO guidelines (2011),* and the *DGGG, OEGGG, SGGG (2020)* all endorse the use of 25 µg of misoprostol for cervical ripening, whether administered orally or vaginally. Similarly, *NICE guidelines (2021)* support the use of low-dose (25 µg) oral misoprostol for labor induction in women with a Bishop score of 6 or less.

ACOG guidelines (2009) suggest an initial dose of 25 µg, to be administered every 3–6 hours, while *WHO guidelines (2011)* recommend oral administration every 2 hours or vaginal administration every 6 hours.

DGGG, OEGGG, SGGG guidelines (2020) additionally note that an oral dose of 50 mcg is considered equivalent in safety to a vaginal dose of 25 µg. *ACOG guidelines (2009)* caution against the use of higher doses, such as 50 mcg every 6 hours, due to the increased risks of uterine tachysystole and fetal heart rate decelerations. Furthermore, both *ACOG guidelines (2009) and WHO guidelines (2011)* recommend avoiding misoprostol in women with a previous cesarean delivery or major uterine surgery because of the heightened risk of uterine rupture. *FOGSI-ICOG GCPR (2018)* also notes that misoprostol has not been approved for labor induction by the Drug Controller General of India, while the *SLCOG (2013)* and the *Queensland guidelines (2022)* advise against its use for labor induction in cases involving a live fetus.

Q4. How does balloon catheter compare with dinoprostone (PGE2) and misoprostol (PGE1) as regards effectiveness and safety for cervical ripening?

Draft recommendations: Mechanical method (balloon catheter) is preferred over prostaglandins for cervical ripening in certain high-risk conditions method in grand multipara/SGA or FGR/oligohydramnios or previously scarred uterus compared to prostaglandins.

Evidence summary:
Balloon Catheter versus Dinoprostone: NICE guidelines (2015) recommend that the use of a balloon catheter for cervical ripening is associated with a significantly lower incidence of uterine tachysystole compared to dinoprostone gel, particularly in cases with an unripe cervix and oligohydramnios. The *FOGSI-ICOG GCPR (2018)* and *Polish guidelines (2017)* reiterate that cervical ripening with a balloon catheter is a safe, affordable, easy to store and preferred in cases of scarred uterus and unfavorable cervix provided there are no signs of infection. It causes less uterine hyperstimulation as compared to prostaglandins and has a reduced risk of serious neonatal morbidity or perinatal death but does not reduce cesarean rates as compared to dinoprostone.

Balloon catheter versus misoprostol: WHO guidelines (2022) suggest using a balloon catheter with oxytocin as an alternative method where prostaglandins are contraindicated or not available. *Polish guidelines (2017)* state that the use of a balloon catheter for preinduction cervical ripening is a simple and inexpensive method with fewer side effects compared to pharmacological agents like misoprostol. It is particularly recommended in grand multiparity, SGA or FGR, and oligohydramnios over other methods. As per the *Queensland guidelines (2022),* it can be used in outpatient setting.

SOGC guidelines (2023) support the concurrent use of prostaglandins and balloon catheters for cervical ripening.

SPECIAL SITUATIONS

Q1. Which is the preferred method(s) of choice for cervical ripening in pregnant women with preterm or prelabor rupture of membranes?

Draft recommendations:

1. Prostaglandins PGE1 and PGE2 by oral route can be used for cervical ripening in women with preterm or prelabor rupture of membranes.
2. Mechanical methods are not recommended.

Evidence summary: The evidence suggests that prostaglandins (PGE1 and PGE2) are commonly recommended for cervical ripening in women with prelabor rupture of membranes, with guidelines generally supporting their use. *FOGSI-ICOG GCPR (2018)* does not consider the vaginal and intracervical dinoprostone to be very effective in women with ruptured membranes. It recommends dinoprostone vaginal pessary (10 mg, released at 0.3 mg/hour over the 24-hour dosing period), which also does not necessitate its removal even after rupture of membrane. According to the *RCOG scientific impact paper (2022),* the method for cervical ripening in pregnant women with prelabor rupture of membranes involves the use of oral misoprostol and dinoprostone. The use of mechanical methods has not been widely studied in these cases.

Q2. Which is the preferred method(s) of choice for cervical ripening in pregnant women with previous cesarean section?

Draft recommendations:

1. For cervical ripening in women with previous lower segment cesarean section (LSCS), mechanical methods, particularly balloon catheters, are preferred.
2. Prostaglandin E2 (dinoprostone) can be used cautiously with close monitoring, but misoprostol should be avoided.

Evidence summary: When reviewing guidelines on cervical ripening in women with a previous lower segment cesarean section (LSCS), a consistent preference emerges for mechanical methods, particularly balloon catheters, due to their lower associated risk of uterine rupture. This recommendation is supported across multiple guidelines, although specific details and emphases vary. *ACOG guidelines (2009), WHO guidelines (2011), FOGSI-ICOG-GCPR (2018), Queensland guidelines (2020), and NICE guidelines (2021)* all recommend use of mechanical methods over pharmacologic options for cervical ripening in women with prior cesarean deliveries. *WHO guidelines (2011) and FOGSI-ICOG-GCPR (2018)* recommend against using misoprostol due to its associated risks.

However, *DGGG, OEGGG, and SGGG guidelines* emphasize that in woman with previous LSCS and an unripe cervix (Bishop score <6), labor can be induced using prostaglandin E2 (dinoprostone), although there is an increased risk of uterine rupture. Mechanical methods such as transcervical balloon catheter and amniotomy are associated with a lower risk of uterine rupture compared to the use of prostaglandins. It is critical to note that misoprostol must not be used for cervical ripening or labor induction in the third trimester for women who have had a previous cesarean section or any surgery involving the uterine cavity, due to the significantly higher risk of uterine rupture.

Q3. Can more than one method of cervical ripening be used sequentially?

Draft recommendations:

1. Sequential use of cervical ripening methods, such as balloon catheters followed by prostaglandins, can be used with caution.
2. Simultaneous use of multiple methods is not recommended.

Evidence summary: Guidelines on the use of multiple cervical ripening methods provide varying recommendations. *WHO guidelines (2011)* suggest that a combination of balloon catheter and oxytocin may be considered when prostaglandins are unavailable or contraindicate. The *DGGG, OEGGG, and SGGG guidelines (2020)* advocate for sequential use of induction methods, such as starting with balloon catheters followed by prostaglandins, particularly for primiparous women with an unripe cervix. They also support the simultaneous induction of labor using balloon catheters and oxytocin or prostaglandins, which has been shown to be effective and results in a shorter interval between induction and delivery compared to using only one method.

Q4. Can the process of cervical ripening be repeated after a rest period if the cervix remains unfavorable after an initial attempt at cervical ripening?

Draft recommendations: In cases of unsuccessful cervical ripening, a rest period followed by repeat or an alternate method may be considered after a thorough reassessment of the pregnant woman and the fetus.

Good practice point: *The approach must be tailored to the individual circumstances and preferences of the patient, keeping in mind the urgency of the clinical situation.*

Evidence summary: *FOGSI-ICOG-GCPR (2018)* recommends that, after reassessing maternal and fetal wellbeing, another attempt to induce labor with a different method can be considered based on clinical judgment and urgency. **Queensland guidelines** (2020) suggest that cervical ripening can be prolonged if the initial Bishop score is low. They recommend considering further attempts with an alternative method, after a reassessment of maternal and fetal condition and a rest period. This approach highlights individualized care and required continuous fetal monitoring. *RCOG Scientific Impact Paper (2022)* supports changing methods after a 24–48-hour interval or a rest period. It also considers cesarean birth as an option, emphasizing a tailored approach depending on individual circumstances and preferences.

CHAPTER 4

Methods of Induction of Labor

Anubhuti Rana, Tanisha Gupta, Apoorva Kulshrestha

OXYTOCIN

Q1. What is the desired Bishop score for initiating oxytocin infusion for induction of labor?

Draft recommendations: Oxytocin infusion is recommended for induction of labor when the Bishop score >6.

Evidence summary: All major guidelines recommend the use of intravenous oxytocin for labor induction when the bishop score is greater than 6. This is strongly supported by *WHO guidelines (2011), SLCOG guidelines (2013), FOGSI-ICOG-GCPR (2018), DGGG, OEGGG, and SGGG guidelines (2020), NICE guidelines (2021), Queensland guidelines (2022), SOGC guidelines (2023), and ACOG guidelines (2024).*

Q2. Can different methods of induction be used simultaneously with oxytocin?

Draft recommendations: Simultaneous induction with amniotomy and oxytocin, and balloon catheter with oxytocin may be offered to reduce the induction delivery interval.

Evidence summary: Amniotomy combined with oxytocin is recommended by *FOGSI-ICOG-GCPR (2018), DGGG, OEGGG, and SGGG guidelines (2020), NICE guidelines (2021), and SOGC guidelines (2023)*. Both *NICE guidelines (2021) and SOGC guidelines (2023)* strongly recommend performing amniotomy before starting oxytocin. Simultaneous induction with balloon catheters and oxytocin or prostaglandins is recommended by **DGGG,** *OEGGG, and SGGG (2020) guidelines*. It results in a shorter time from induction to delivery compared to using a single method; this combination is also recommended as an alternative method by *WHO guidelines (2011)*.

Q3. What should be the time interval between cervical ripening with prostaglandins and induction of labor with oxytocin?

Draft recommendations: Oxytocin should be administered at least 6 hours after inserting vaginal prostaglandin E2, 30 minutes after removing a prostaglandin E2 vaginal insert, 2 hours after administering oral misoprostol, and 4 hours after inserting vaginal misoprostol.

Evidence summary: The *European Association of Perinatal Medicine guidelines (2021), Queensland guidelines (2022), and SOGC guidelines (2023)* provide specific recommendations for timing oxytocin administration following prostaglandin use. They recommend starting oxytocin no earlier than 30 minutes after removing a prostaglandin E2 vaginal insert, 6 hours after inserting a prostaglandin E2 vaginal gel, 2 hours after administering oral prostaglandin E1, and 4 hours after inserting vaginal prostaglandin E1.

Q4. What are the various methods to titrate oxytocin infusion and how do they compare?

Draft recommendations:

1. Oxytocin should be administered intravenously as an infusion for induction of labor to allow continuous and precise dose control.
   Infusion rates must be recorded in milliunits per minute (mU/min) or drops per minute, with the dilution specified.
2. The standard preparation involves diluting 5U of oxytocin in 500 mL (10 mU/mL) of normal saline or Ringer's lactate solution. Both high-dose and low-dose regimens are recommended in primigravida. The low-dose regimen begins at 1 to 2 mU/min, with incremental increases of 1–2 mU every 30 minutes. The high-dose regimen starts at 4 to 6 mU/min, with increments of 4 to 6 mU/min every 15–30 minutes.
3. High-dose regimens are not recommended for multigravida and women with a previously scarred uterus.

Evidence summary: Oxytocin infusion protocols for labor induction and augmentation vary widely, primarily because there is no predictable dose response for uterine contractions. Each facility should develop specific protocols for the preparation and administration of oxytocin. Oxytocin should be administered intravenously as an infusion to allow continuous and precise control over the dose. Infusion rates should be documented in milliunits per minute (mU/min) or drops per minute, with the dilution specified. For fluid selection, isotonic solutions such as Ringer's lactate or normal saline are preferred over dextrose solutions to minimize the risk of electrolyte imbalance (e.g., hyponatremia) and volume overload, as recommended by *SLCOG guidelines (2014), Safer Care Victoria guidelines (2017), FOGSI-ICOG-GCPR (2018), and the European Association of Perinatal Medicine guidelines (2021), ACOG guidelines (2024).* Most guidelines recommend a dilution of 10 units of oxytocin in 1 liter of solution (5 U in 500 mL), except for *WHO guidelines (2007),* which recommend starting with a dilution of 2.5 units of oxytocin in 500 mL of solution.

FOGSI-ICOG-GCPR (2018) and *ACOG guidelines (2024)* support using both high- and low-dose infusion protocols. The low-dose regimen begins with 1–2 mU/min, with incremental increases of 1–2 mU every 30 minutes.

The high-dose regimen starts with 4–6 mU/min, with increments of 4–6 mU/min every 15–30 minutes.

WHO guidelines (2007) recommend starting at 10 drops/min (2.5 units in 500 mL), approximately 2.5 mU/min, and increasing by 10 drops per minute every 30 minutes until a good contraction pattern is established, up to a maximum of 60 drops per minute (15 mU/min). If a good contraction pattern is not established at 60 drops per minute, the oxytocin concentration is increased to 5 units in 500 mL of normal saline, starting at 30 drops per minute (15 mU/min), with increments of 10 drops per minute every 30 minutes until a good contraction pattern is established or the maximum rate of 60 drops per minute is reached (30 mU/min). In primigravida, further increases can be made. For higher concentration (10 units in 500 mL), oxytocin is started at 15 drops per minute, with increases every 15 minutes to a maximum of 60 drops per minute (60 mU/min). It is suggested not to use oxytocin 10 units in 500 mL (i.e., 20 mU/mL) in multigravida and women with previous cesarean section. Rapid escalation by 15 drops/min is also not advised in multigravida and scarred uterus. According to *SLCOG guidelines (2014)*, 5 units in 500 mL oxytocin is administered starting at a drop rate of 15 drops per minute, equivalent to 7.5 mU/min, and increased by 15 drops per minute every 30 minutes, up to a maximum of 60 drops per minute (30 mU/min). When using infusion pumps, oxytocin is prepared at 10 units in 500 mL, with a starting dose of 1 mU/min at a rate of 3 mL/h, escalated every 30 minutes as needed. *NICE guidelines (2021)* recommend that the time between dose increments should be no more frequent than every 30 minutes.

Titration should be done according to the contraction pattern, with all guidelines advising titration until good contractions are established (three contractions in 10 minutes, each lasting more than 40 seconds). This rate should be maintained until delivery. Oxytocin should be stopped or reduced if contractions occur more frequently than 4–5 in 10 minutes.

Q5. What is the maximum recommended dose of oxytocin in mU/min for induction of labor in primigravidae and multigravidae?

Draft recommendations: A maximum dose of 60 mU/min of oxytocin is recommended for primigravidae while a maximum of 30 mU/min for multigravidae and women with a previous cesarean section.

Evidence summary: *WHO guidelines (2007)* recommend a maximum dose of 60 mU/min for primigravida and 30 mU/min for multigravida and women with a scarred uterus. *SLCOG guidelines (2014)* suggest a maximum dose of 30 mU/min and *FOGSI-ICOG-GCPR (2018)* advises an upper limit of 40 mU/min during labor with a live fetus in the third trimester (GCPR). *NICE guidelines (2021)* and *ACOG guidelines (2024)* do not specify any maximum dose.

MISOPROSTOL

Q1. What are the various routes and doses of misoprostol for induction of labor?

Draft recommendations:

1. For the induction of labor, misoprostol may be administered by oral, sublingual, or vaginal route.
2. A dose of a 25 μg misoprostol is recommended every 2 hours for oral route and every 6 hours for vaginal route. The dose should be titrated based on the frequency and duration of uterine contractions.
3. Misoprostol is not recommended for induction of labor in a scarred uterus.

Evidence summary: The use of misoprostol for induction of labor varies across guidelines. The *WHO guidelines (2011), DGGG, OEGGG,* and *SGGG guidelines (2020), SOGC guidelines (2023)* recommend misoprostol for induction of labor. In contrast, *ACOG guidelines (2009)* and *NICE guidelines (2021)* recommend it only for cervical ripening, and the *Queensland guidelines (2022)* and *SLCOG guidelines (2013)* do not recommend misoprostol for induction of labor with a live fetus.

Misoprostol can be administered orally, vaginally, buccally, or sublingually. The pharmacokinetics vary. Oral and sublingual routes peak at about 30 minutes, while buccal and vaginal administration peak at 70–80 minutes. Oral misoprostol has a half-life of 20–40 minutes with a duration of action of 2 hours, whereas with vaginal administration action lasts around 4 hours. *WHO guidelines (2011)* recommend oral administration at 25 μg every 2 hours and vaginal administration at 25 μg every 6 hours and *DGGG, OEGGG, and SGGG guidelines (2020)* recommend both administration of misoprostol by both oral (50 μg) and vaginal (25 μg) routes. *The SOGC guidelines (2023)* recommend starting with 20–25 μg of oral misoprostol, titrated to contractions, with a maximum dose of less than 50 μg.

AMNIOTOMY

Q1. When should amniotomy be done during the induction of labor?

Draft recommendations: Amniotomy is recommended for labor induction when the Bishop score is ≥6, and should be used in combination with oxytocin infusion depending on intensity of uterine contraction.

Evidence summary: *ACOG guidelines (2009), WHO guidelines (2011), SLGOC guidelines (2013), FOGSI-ICOG-GCPR (2018), DGGG, OEGGG and SGGG guidelines (2020), Queensland guidelines (2022), NICE guidelines (2021) and SOGC guidelines (2023)* all recommend use of amniotomy for induction of labor after cervical ripening (Bishop's score >6). All the guidelines recommend combining oxytocin with amniotomy if there are inadequate contractions.

MIFEPRISTONE

Q1. What are the indication, dose, and route for mifepristone for induction of labor?

Draft recommendations:

1. Due to insufficient evidence, mifepristone is not currently recommended for inducing labor in live pregnancies.
2. In women with intrauterine fetal demise, oral dose of 200–600 mg per day for 1–2 days can be used for cervical ripening.

Evidence summary: Currently, no guidelines recommend using mifepristone for inducing labor in live pregnancies. However, mifepristone, a progesterone antagonist, is known to cause softening and dilation of the cervix in early pregnancy and increase uterine activity. Because of these effects, mifepristone may be a valuable agent for cervical ripening and labor induction. Several studies have explored its use for this purpose. A 2009 Cochrane analysis of 10 clinical trials involving 1,108 patients compared mifepristone to a placebo for labor induction. Patients who received mifepristone were significantly more likely to have a favorable cervix at 48 hours (RR 2.41; 95% CI 1.70–3.42), were less likely to require oxytocin augmentation (RR 0.80; 95% CI 0.66–0.97), and had a lower likelihood of needing a cesarean delivery due to failed induction (RR 0.40; 95% CI 0.20–0.80) than those given a placebo. According to the authors' analysis, a single 200 mg oral dose of mifepristone seems to be the minimum effective dose for cervical ripening, with optimal effects observed at 72 hours. *RCOG guidelines (2010), DGGG, OEGGG and SGGG guidelines (2020), and NICE guidelines (2021)* recommend 600 mg daily for two days orally and *FIGO guidelines (2023)* suggest a 200 mg single dose for inducing labor in cases of intrauterine demise.

BIBLIOGRAPHY

1. ACOG Practice Bulletin No. 107: Induction of labor. Obstet Gynecol. 2009;114 (2 Pt 1):386-97.
2. ACOG Practice Bulletin No. 190 Summary: Gestational Diabetes Mellitus. Obstet & Gynecol. 2018;131(2):406-8.
3. Berger H, Gagnon R, Sermer M. Guideline No. 393-Diabetes in Pregnancy. J Obstet Gynaecol Can. 2019;41(12):1814-25.e1.
4. Boers KE, Vijgen SMC, Bijlenga D, et al. Induction versus expectant monitoring for intrauterine growth restriction at term: randomised equivalence trial (DIGITAT). BMJ. 2010;341:c7087.
5. Bomba-Opoń D, Drews K, Huras H, et al. Polish Gynecological Society Recommendations for Labor Induction. Ginekol Pol. 2017;88(4):224-34.
6. Borovac-Pinheiro A, Inversetti A, Di Simone N, et al; FIGO Childbirth and Postpartum Hemorrhage Committee. FIGO good practice recommendations for induced or spontaneous labor at term: Prep-for-Labor triage to minimize

risks and maximize favorable outcomes. Int J Gynaecol Obstet. 2023;163 (Suppl 2):51-6.

7. Delaney M, Roggensack A. No. 214-Guidelines for the Management of Pregnancy at 41+0 to 42+0 Weeks. J Obstet Gynaecol Can. 2017;39(8):e164-74.
8. Editor T. Guideline for use of oxytocin for induction and augmentation of labour. Sri Lanka J Obstet Gynae. 2014;35(4):139.
9. Editor T. Guideline on induction of labour. Sri Lanka J Obstet Gynae. 2014; 35(4):136.
10. FIGO. (2023). FIGO Mifepristone & Misoprostol and Misoprostol Only Dosing Charts 2023. [online] Available from: https://www.figo.org/figo-mifepristone-misoprostol-and-misoprostol-only-dosing-charts-2023 [Last accessed November, 2024].
11. First and Second Stage Labor Management: ACOG Clinical Practice Guideline No. 8. Obstet Gynecol. 2024;143(1):144–62.
12. FOGSI-ICOG. (2018) Good clinical practice recommendations. [online] Available from: https://www.fogsi.org/wp-content/uploads/2018/09/XGCPR-IOL-26July.pdf [Last accessed November, 2024].
13. Gestational Hypertension and Preeclampsia: ACOG Practice Bulletin Summary, Number 222. Obstet Gynecol. 2020;135(6):1492–5.
14. Girling J, Knight CL, Chappell L; the Royal College of Obstetricians and Gynaecologists. Intrahepatic cholestasis of pregnancy: Green-top Guideline No. 43 June 2022. BJOG. 2022;129(13):e95-e114.
15. Grobman WA, Rice MM, Reddy UM, et al. Labor Induction versus Expectant Management in Low-risk Nulliparous Women. N Engl J Med. 2018;379(6): 513-23.
16. Hagenbeck C, Hamza A, Kehl S, et al. Management of Intrahepatic Cholestasis of Pregnancy: Recommendations of the Working Group on Obstetrics and Prenatal Medicine - Section on Maternal Disorders. Geburtshilfe Frauenheilkd. 2021;81(8):922-39.
17. Hague WM, Briley A, Callaway L, et al. Intrahepatic cholestasis of pregnancy—Diagnosis and management: a consensus statement of the Society of Obstetric Medicine of Australia and New Zealand (SOMANZ): Executive Summary. Aust NZ J Obst Gynaeco. 2023;63(5):656-65.
18. Hapangama D, Neilson JP. Mifepristone for induction of labour. Cochrane Database Syst Rev. 2009;2009(3):CD002865.
19. Infant wellbeing at 2 years of age in the Growth Restriction Intervention Trial (GRIT): multicentred randomised controlled trial. Lancet. 2004;364(9433): 513-20.
20. Kehl S, Hösli I, Pecks U, et al. Induction of Labour. Guideline of the DGGG, OEGGG and SGGG (S2k, AWMF Registry No. 015-088, December 2020). Geburtshilfe Frauenheilkd. 2021;81(8):870-95.
21. Lee HS, Abbasi N, Van Mieghem T, et al. Guideline No. 440: Management of Monochorionic Twin Pregnancies. J Obstet Gynaecol Can. 2023;45(8): 587-606.e8.
22. Lees CC, Marlow N, Van Wassenaer-Leemhuis A, et al. 2-year neurodevelopmental and intermediate perinatal outcomes in infants with very preterm fetal growth restriction (TRUFFLE): a randomised trial. Lancet. 2015;385(9983): 2162-72.

23. Lees CC, Stampalija T, Baschat A, et al. ISUOG Practice Guidelines: diagnosis and management of small-for-gestational-age fetus and fetal growth restriction. Ultrasound Obstet Gynecol. 2020;56(2):298-312.
24. Magee LA, Smith GN, Bloch C, et al. Guideline No. 426: Hypertensive Disorders of Pregnancy: Diagnosis, Prediction, Prevention, and Management. J Obstetr Gynaecol Can. 2022;44(5):547-71.e1.
25. Managing Complication in Pregnancy and Childbirth: A Guide for Midwives and Doctors, 2nd edited. Geneva, Switzerland: World Health Organization; 2017.
26. Mei-Dan E, Jain V, Melamed N, et al. Guideline No. 428: Management of Dichorionic Twin Pregnancies. J Obstet Gynaecol Can. 2022;44(7):819-34.e1.
27. Melamed N, Baschat A, Yinon Y, et al. FIGO (International Federation of Gynecology and Obstetrics) initiative on fetal growth: Best practice advice for screening, diagnosis, and management of fetal growth restriction. Intl J Gynecology Obste. 2021;152(S1):3-57.
28. Metz TD, Berry RS, Fretts RC, et al. Obstetric Care Consensus #10: Management of Stillbirth. Am J Obstet Gynecol. 2020;222(3):B2-20.
29. Ministry of health and Family welfare India. (2018). Diagnosis and Management of gestational diabetes mellitus. Technical operational guidelines. [online] Available from: https://nhm.gov.in/New_Updates_2018/NHM_Components/RMNCH_MH_Guidelines/Gestational-Diabetes-Mellitus.pdf [Last accessed November, 2024].
30. Morris RK, Johnstone E, Lees C, et al; the Royal College of Obstetricians and Gynaecologists. Investigation and Care of a SMALL-FOR-GESTATIONAL-AGE Fetus and a Growth Restricted Fetus (Green-top Guideline No. 31). BJOG. 2024;131(9).
31. Multifetal Gestations: Twin, Triplet, and Higher-Order Multifetal Pregnancies: ACOG Practice Bulletin, Number 231. Obstetr Gynecol. 2021;137(6):e145-62.
32. National Institute for Health and Care Excellence (NICE). (2024). Twin and triplet pregnancy. (NICE Guideline, No. 137). [online] Available from: https://www.ncbi.nlm.nih.gov/books/NBK546070/ [Last accessed November, 2024].
33. NICE. (2015). Insertion of a double balloon catheter for induction of labour in pregnant women without previous caesarean section. [online] Available from: https://www.nice.org.uk/guidance/ipg528 [Last accessed November, 2024].
34. NICE. (2015). NICE guideline [NG3] Diabetes in pregnancy: management from preconception to the postnatal period. [online] Available from: https://www.nice.org.uk/guidance/ng3 [Last accessed November, 2024].
35. NICE. (2019). Hypertension in pregnancy: diagnosis and management NICE guideline [NG133]. [online] Available from: https://www.nice.org.uk/guidance/ng133/ [Last accessed November, 2024].
36. NICE. (2021). NICE guideline {NG 207] induction of labor. [online]. Available from: https://www.nice.org.uk/guidance/ng207 [Last accessed November, 2024].
37. NICE. (2022). NICE guideline 229. Fetal monitoring in labour. [Online] Available from https://www.nice.org.uk/guidance/ng229/resources/fetal-monitoring-in-labour-pdf-66143844065221 [Last accessed November, 2024].

38. NICE. (2023). NICE guideline [NG235] Intrapartum care. [online] Available from: https://www.nice.org.uk/guidance/ng235 [Last accessed November, 2024].
39. Obstetric care consensus no. 1: safe prevention of the primary cesarean delivery. Obstet Gynecol. 2014;123(3):693-711.
40. Queensland Clinical Guidelines. (2022). Gestational diabetes mellitus (GDM). Guideline No. MN21.33-V6-R26. Queensland Health. [online] Available from: http://health.qld.gov.au/qcg [Last accessed November, 2024].
41. Queensland Clinical Guidelines. (2022). Induction of labour. Guideline No. MN22.22-V9-R27. Queensland Health. [online] Available from: http://www.health.qld.gov.au/qcg [Last accessed November, 2024].
42. RCOG. (2010). Care of late intrauterine fetal death and still birth. [online] Available from: https://www.rcog.org.uk/guidance/browse-all-guidance/green-top-guidelines/late-intrauterine-fetal-death-and-stillbirth-green-top-guideline-no-55/ [Last accessed November, 2024].
43. Robinson D, Campbell K, Hobson SR, et al. Guideline No. 432b: Cervical Ripening. J Obstet Gynaecol Can. 2023;45(1):56-62.e1.
44. Robinson D, Campbell K, Hobson SR, et al. Guideline No. 432c: Induction of Labour. J Obstet Gynaecol Can. 2023;45(1):70-77.e3.
45. Ryberg J, Carlsson Y, Svensson M, et al. Risk of uterine rupture in multiparous women after induction of labor with prostaglandin: a national population-based cohort study. Int J Gynaecol Obstet. 2024;165(1):328-34.
46. Saccone G, Della Corte L, Maruotti GM, et al. Induction of labor at full-term in pregnant women with uncomplicated singleton pregnancy: a systematic review and meta-analysis of randomized trials. Acta Obstet Gynecol Scand. 2019;98(8):958-66.
47. Safer Care Victoria. (2017). Induction of labor. [online] Available from: https://www.safercare.vic.gov.au/best-practice-improvement/clinical-guidance/maternity/induction-of-labour [Last accessed November, 2024].
48. Sotiriadis A, Petousis S, Thilaganathan B, et al. Maternal and perinatal outcomes after elective induction of labor at 39 weeks in uncomplicated singleton pregnancy: a meta-analysis. Ultrasound Obstet Gynecol. 2019;53(1):26-35.
49. Weeks AD, Lightly K, Mol BW, et al. Evaluating misoprostol and mechanical methods for induction of labour: Scientific Impact Paper No. 68 April 2022. BJOG. 2022;129(8).
50. WHO. (2000). Managing Complications in Pregnancy and Childbirth: A guide for midwives and doctors. [online] Available from: https://iris.who.int/bitstream/handle/10665/43972/9241545879_eng.pdf;sequence=1 [Last accessed November, 2024].
51. WHO. (2011). WHO recommendations on induction of labor. [online] Available from: https://iris.who.int/bitstream/handle/10665/44531/9789241501156_eng.pdf?sequence=1 [Last accessed November, 2024].
52. WHO. (2018). WHO recommendations for augmentation of labor. [online] Available from: https://iris.who.int/bitstream/handle/10665/112825/9789241507363_eng.pdf?sequence=1 [Last accessed November, 2024].
53. WHO. (2022). WHO recommendations for induction of labor at or beyond term. [online] Available from: https://iris.who.int/bitstream/

handle/10665/363138/9789240052796-eng.pdf?sequence=1 [Last accessed November, 2024].

54. WHO. (2022). WHO recommendations on mechanical methods for induction of labour. [online] Available from: https://iris.who.int/bitstream/handle/10665/363140/9789240055780-eng.pdf?sequence=1 [Last accessed November, 2024].
55. Writing group; Nunes I, Dupont C, Timonen S, et al. European Guidelines on Perinatal Care - Oxytocin for induction and augmentation of labor. J Matern Fetal Neonat Med. 2024;35(25):7166-72.